Table of Contents

INTRODUCTION

Anyone who has ever tried to lose weight on their own knows: It's no walk in the park. But with so many diet companies claiming to have cracked the code on weight loss, choosing the best diet plan can feel even harder. The truth is, there is no miracle one-size-fits-all weight loss plan, and the best diet plan for weight loss is the one you can actually stick with. That means it's important to decide what you value most in a diet plan, and base your selection on that. The SparkDiet is a four-stage process that teaches you how to get over the dieting hump. Built on motivation and momentum, the SparkDiet helps you make the transition from dieting to living a healthy lifestyle where you don’t need to diet anymore. Through regular action steps, the diet program walks you through smart weight loss strategies designed to eliminate yo-yo results. Read on to learn more about this diet.

CHAPTER ONE

What Is Spark Solution Diet?

The folks behind the online diet and healthy-living community SparkPeople.com believe the Spark Solution diet will help you lose weight as a result of nutritious, reduced-calorie meal plans that optimize your metabolism. According to the plan, two weeks of structured diet and exercise will put you on the fast track to successful weight loss and healthier living. You'll also complement the diet with regular fitness and maintain momentum with positive reinforcement and advice from people who've benefited from the Spark Solution. The 1,500-calorie diet breaks down to 45 to 65 percent carbohydrates, 20 to 35 percent fats and 16 to 35 percent proteins. Meal plans include breakfast, lunch, dinner and snacks, and the diet guidebook provides specific recipes. These meals are dubbed "Spark Swaps" and are pitted against typical, less healthy meals. For example, instead of snacking on 1 ounce of potato chips on day one, the meal plan proposes making a healthy swap for 12 almonds. The book shows how many calories the swap saves, why the swap is a healthier choice and other nutrition tips.

How Does Spark Solution Diet Work?

Dieters follow "The Spark Solution" book, which gives detailed guidance for the meal plan's first two weeks. You can download the free SparkPeople Calorie Calculator and Diet Tracker app to find healthy recipes, look up nutrition information for more than 3 million foods, track activity and more. Here are some tips for getting started on Spark food swaps:

- Substitute quinoa for brown rice.
- Breakfast with traditional or steel-cut oatmeal instead of cold cereal.

- Use Greek yogurt to substitute for sour cream when cooking.
- Select kale or spinach rather than romaine lettuce for added nutrition.
- Choose sweet potatoes, not white potatoes, to add vitamins and reduce blood-sugar spikes.

Daily, you'll eat three to four servings of raw or cooked nonstarchy vegetables. Two to three servings of fruit – fresh, frozen or canned – are part of the plan. You'll also include five to six servings of whole grains and starchy vegetables combined. You'll incorporate protein with two to three servings of lean, low-fat animal meat or plant-based proteins. You can have two daily servings each of dairy and fats, as part of a meal or in snacks. Exercise plays a significant role in the Spark Solution. In addition to meal plans, the book provides daily workouts for the first two weeks. Roughly 40 pages are devoted to fitness, including photos to show how certain exercises should be performed, a workout "menu" detailing the number of calories various workouts burn and other practical fitness guidance. Followers can access fitness coaching and advice via the app, too. Each day, dieters also read about the mental aspects of dieting in a series called the "Mind-Set Makeover." Dieters might, for example, learn about stress eating and tips for relaxing. Each day's plan concludes with a daily reflection. The diet authors figure it takes about two weeks to create and maintain healthy diets and point out that many people fall off the diet wagon in the first two weeks. While the book provides follow-up guidance for weeks three, four and beyond, detailed meal plans and exercise routines are provided for the first 14 days.

What Types Of Meals Should I Eat On Spark Solution Diet?

A little bit of everything, given that Spark Solution meal plans are pretty well-rounded. Each day, you're eating three to four servings of nonstarchy vegetables, typically raw or cooked, and two to three servings of fruit, either fresh, frozen or canned (but not in that heavy syrup). You'll also eat five to six servings of whole grains and starchy vegetables, as well as two to three servings of protein in the form of lean, low-fat animal meat or plant-based proteins. You're allotted two daily servings each of dairy and fats on the Spark Solution, either with a meal or via snacks.

Will Spark Solution Diet Help Me Lose Weight?

The Spark Solution diet will probably help you lose weight. If you successfully stick to the plan, you'll be exercising regularly and limiting your calories to about 1,500 per day – a combination that's likely to drop a few pounds. At this point, little research specifically examines the Spark Solution. However, studies that look at the effects of the Spark Solution's two broad tenets – diet and weight loss – provide some insight.

- A 2009 study published in Obesity Reviews compared the weight-loss successes of people who dieted and exercised versus those who only dieted. The researchers found that participants who both dieted and exercised had greater long-term weight loss.
- A 2012 study in the journal Obesity looked at weight loss interventions for obese and overweight sedentary postmenopausal women.

While the control group maintained their lifestyles, a second group adopted a reduced-calorie low-fat diet, a third group began an exercise program and the fourth group tried a combination of both diet and exercise interventions. After a year, the dieters lost an average of 16 pounds; the exercisers lost an average of 4 1/2 pounds; and the group that combined diet and exercise lost an average of nearly 20 pounds.

How Easy Is Spark Solution Diet To Follow?

The Spark Solution will likely work best for people who enjoy planning and do well with structure. If that doesn't sound like you, the diet's detailed guidelines and rules may be tough to digest. This plan will also keep you from dining out for the first few weeks, and it's impractical for folks who are unable to (or simply won't) exercise regularly.

- The diet gives you specific directions. The Spark Solution guidelines are specific, which makes it convenient for dieters who don't want to make any decisions, but perhaps a pain for others.

- New recipes are encouraged. For the first three weeks, dieters are supposed to follow the recipes and meal plans found in the "The Spark Solution" book. At week four, dieters can "spark it up" by adding recipes that aren't in the book, so long as they follow the Spark Solution guidelines for calories, protein, fats and carbs. The authors suggest finding recipes and nutritional information for various foods on SparkRecipes.com or via the Healthy Recipes app.
- Eating out is possible. Dining out becomes an option in week four of the Spark Solution, as long as dieters continue to abide by their nutritional goals, track their food intake and measure portions. Menus with nutritional information will eliminate much of the guesswork when eating out.
- Plan your meals ahead with help. Not many timesavers are available, unless you hire somebody to plan, shop for and prepare your

meals. However, the Spark Solution provides tips for planning ahead on the next day's meals. Followers can also sync the Healthy Recipes app with the Calorie Counter and Diet Tracker app so they don't have to track their calories manually.

- Spark Solution offers extras. SparkPeople.com includes a Spark Solution forum to connect with other dieters, and SparkRecipes.com and the Healthy Recipes app offer hundreds of thousands of healthy recipes. The SparkPeople Calorie Counter and Diet Tracker also offers video demos by professional chefs and a conversion calculator in case you need to figure out, say, how many cups are in a liter. For added motivation, the website's Challenge Central offers two types of momentum-building programs, including calendar challenges like the '5K Your Way" walk/jog challenge.
- Feeling full shouldn't be a problem. Nutrition experts emphasize the importance of satiety, or the satisfied feeling that you've had enough. While you'll consume fewer calories than the

average American, the Spark Solution meal plans include breakfast, lunch, dinner and snacks, which should help to curb hunger. The meal plan analyzed above also provides a whopping 38 grams of fiber, which may help you feel fuller for a longer period of time.

- Taste is up to you. If you don't love what's on tap for that day's meal plan, then it's up to you to tweak the ingredients to make meals more enjoyable.

How Much Should I Exercise On Spark Solution Diet?

Exercise is key to the Spark Solution diet. Along with daily workouts for the first two weeks, the book provides roughly 40 pages devoted to fitness, including photos to show how certain exercises should be performed, a workout "menu" with the number of calories various workouts burn and other practical fitness guidance. The app also offers fitness guidance; those on the premium plan can email coaches questions about their routines.

What Are The Pros And Cons Of The Spark Solution Diet?

A balanced diet that resembles the Flexitarian diet and the Mayo Clinic Diet, the Spark Solution is a popular diet that promises impressive results in just two weeks, followed by consistent weight loss, through a combination of calorie restrictions and exercise.

Pros of the Spark Solution Diet

With just 1,500 calorie per day and plenty of exercise, the Spark Solution can certainly you lose weight, but before committing to its two week plan, followed by additional guidelines. Unlike other diets that promise results in just two weeks, the Spark Solution is nutritionally sound in almost every way. When it comes to daily calories that come from protein, carbs and fat, the diet plan doesn't stray from the government recommendations, and it excels when it comes to calcium intake, a mineral that can aid in weight loss.

It's Structured with Little Room for Error

If you aren't a fan of diet that leave many of the choices up to you, the Spark Solution might prove of great help.

The daily meal plans are specific for the first 14 days, and include plenty of guidelines for sustainable weight loss. The book offers essential information that explains every choice and makes dieting easy.

Keeping your daily calorie intake at around 1,500 and exercising will definitely provide results and the diet can be followed by most people without any difficulty. As long as you stick to the recommendations for the third and fourth week and turn them into a long term plan, you're not likely to gain back the extra pounds.

With around 38 grams of fiber in the sample meal plan, the Sparks Solution diet won't leave you feeling hungry. By getting a healthy dose of fiber, spread out between three daily meals and snacks, the diet promotes satiety. While dieters who want to remain Gluten-free can easily tweak the diet to avoid any wheat and other cereal that contains gluten, vegetarians and vegans might have to work a bit more to adapt it. The Sparks Solution book doesn't offer too many tips for replacing animal protein, but if you've already transitioned to a diet with less meat, you'll be able to make the necessary submissions without a lot of trouble.If you'd like to try new recipes or get advice from other dieters who follow the Spark Solution diet, you'll find an active community at SparkPeople.com and a lot of recipe ideas at SparkRecipes.com.

Cons of the Spark Solution Diet

Dieters who can't prepare all of their meals won't find the Spark Solution particularly attractive, and those with a sedentary lifestyle might be disappointed to learn that fitness plays a big part in the diet.

Lacks Convenience and Options for Eating Out

Since the Spark Solution is very specific, you'll have to plan all of your meals for the first three weeks on the diet. Eating out only becomes an option later, so the structure may not be convenient for dieters who lack the time and patience to follow instructions to the letter.

Includes a Lot of Sodium

If you're not careful, the Sparks Solution may end up increasing your daily sodium intake. While the recommendations vary from a maximum between 1,500 and 2,300 mg, a sample menu can easily push your daily intake over 3,000.

Exercise Is Important

The Sparks Solution book includes detailed workouts for the first couple of weeks and encourages you to exercise in order to lose weight faster. The 1,500 calorie daily limit may leave you without the energy you need to exercise, but the fitness section of the Sparks Solution is designer to appeal to beginners, just like the clear dietary guidelines.

Stages Of Spark Diet

Stage 1: Fast Break (2 Weeks)

- Build the skills and discipline you need by practicing, learning and preparing.
- Focus on a few simple goals to get your mind and body ready.
- Learn to use the meal planner and nutrition tracker, and organize your surroundings.

Stage 2: Healthy Diet Habits (6 Weeks)

- Make specific changes and learn a lot about making smart decisions.
- Learn a new healthy habit each week, along with practical actions steps to carry it out.

- Get more involved with the SparkPeople community and build confidence.
- Habits include: Control Portions; Eat The Right Stuff; Exercise Consistently; Drink Water; Eat On Purpose; Find Unexpected Opportunities

Stage 3: Lifestyle Change (10 Weeks)

- Make that elusive transition from "being on a diet" to "living a fresh new healthy lifestyle."
- Learn how to keep yourself motivated and consistent and use those skills to take your diet – and your life – to another level.

  Strategies include: following your main motivation; involving others; using rewards; bouncing back from setbacks; and dealing with emotional eating.

Stage 4: Spread The Spark (Ongoing)

- With more energy, confidence and motivation, you can pursue goals and dreams in all areas of your life!
- Help others accomplish their own weight loss and healthy living goals.

- Stay engaged through regular "checkups" that evaluate how well you've been sticking to your new healthy lifestyle.

Spark Solution Diet Meal Plan

Here's a sample 1,569-calorie day of meals in the first week of the diet, provided by "The Spark Solution" book.

Breakfast

Spinach-Feta Breakfast Wrap (1 serving):

- 17-inch whole wheat tortilla
- 1/4 cup sliced mushrooms
- 1/4 teaspoon black pepper
- 2 cups (about 6 ounces) fresh spinach
- 1 large egg plus 1 egg white, lightly whisked
- 2 tablespoons crumbled low-fat feta cheese

Lunch

Chicken Caesar Salad (1 serving):

Dressing:

- 1 small clove garlic, minced
- 1/8 teaspoon Dijon mustard
- 1/2 teaspoon miso paste

- 2 teaspoons lemon juice
- 2 tablespoons fat-free plain Greek yogurt

Salad:

- 2 cups Romaine lettuce, chopped or torn into bite-size pieces
- 3 ounces cooked chicken breast, diced
- 1 teaspoon shredded Parmesan cheese
- Pinch of black pepper
- 1 slice whole-wheat bread, toasted and cubed
- 1/2 cup grape or cherry tomatoes
- 16 seedless grapes
- 1 carton (6 ounces) light flavored yogurt

Snack

Avocado toast:

- 1 slice whole-wheat bread, toasted
- 1/4 avocado, mashed
- Black pepper to taste

Dinner

Inside-Out Burgers (4 servings):

- 1 pound 96-percent lean ground beef
- 1 teaspoon black pepper
- 1 small white or yellow onion, cut into four slices
- 1 teaspoon fresh thyme
- 2 teaspoons balsamic vinegar
- 4 whole-wheat Arnold Sandwich Thins, toasted
- 1 large tomato (3-inch diameter), cut into 4 slices
- 4 large lettuce leaves

Baked Garlic Herb Fries (4 servings):

- 1 pound fingerling potatoes (about 12), thinly sliced
- 2 cloves garlic, sliced
- 1 teaspoon minced fresh rosemary
- 1 teaspoon fresh thyme leaves
- 1 cup skim milk

Snack

Berry Cobbler Cup:

- 1 1/2 tablespoons skim milk

- 1 1/2 tablespoons whole-wheat flour
- 2 teaspoons sugar
- 1/4 teaspoon baking powder
- 1/3 cup fresh or frozen berries (blueberries, blackberries and raspberries)

CHAPTER TWO

Spark Diet Recipes

Carribean Brown Rice

Ingredients

- 1 Cup Brown Rice
- 2 Cups Chicken Broth (fat free is best)
- 2 tbls Honey
- 1/4 tsp ground Ginger
- 1/2 tsp ground cinnamon
- Red Pepper flakes to taste (very few -less than 1/4 tsp- make this fairly spicy!)

Directions

For Slightly Firm Rice:

Soak brown rice for 45 minutes in chicken broth. Bring to a boil with a lid on the pot, let simmer until large starchy bubbles begin to come out of the rice, then turn off the heat. Let rice stand with lid on the pot for another 20 minutes. Fold in all the remaining ingredients and serve.

For a Softer, stickier Rice:

Soak rice in broth for 45 min. Bring to boil, when large starchy bubbles come out of rice...add another cup of chicken broth and simmer on med heat for another 20 minutes. Fold in remaining ingredients and serve.

Each serving is approximately 1/3 cup.

Number of Servings: 4

Asparagus Casserole

Ingredients

- cooking spray
- 2 pounds fresh asparagus, trimmed

- ⅔ cup gluten-free bread crumbs
- 2 tablespoons nutritional yeast
- salt and ground black pepper to taste
- 1 cup raw cashews
- 1 cup chicken broth
- ¼ cup nutritional yeast
- ¾ teaspoon garlic powder
- ⅛ teaspoon ground nutmeg
- 1 egg white
- 2 tablespoons bacon bits
- 2 tablespoons sliced almonds
- 2 teaspoons dairy-free margarine, melted

Directions

Preheat the oven to 350 degrees F (175 degrees C). Spray a 7 x 11-inch baking dish with cooking spray. Place a steamer insert into a saucepan and fill with water to just below the bottom of the steamer. Bring water to a boil. Add asparagus, cover, and steam until fork-tender, about 5 minutes. Drain. Combine bread crumbs and 2 tablespoons nutritional yeast in a bowl. Sprinkle 1/2 of the bread crumb mixture on the bottom of the prepared baking dish; top with asparagus spears and season lightly with salt. Reserve remaining bread crumbs for the topping. Combine raw cashews, chicken broth, 1/4 cup nutritional yeast, garlic, nutmeg, salt, and pepper in the bowl of a small food processor or blender. Blend at medium-high speed until mixture is smooth, about 3 minutes. Add egg white and blend at medium-high speed for 1 more minute. Spread blended contents evenly over the asparagus spears, and top with bacon, sliced almonds, and reserved bread crumbs. Drizzle melted margarine over the top. Bake in the preheated oven on the center rack until top is lightly browned and casserole has set, about 30 minutes.

Note:

You can also use crumbled bacon instead of bacon bits.

Meringue Christmas Cookies

Ingredients

- 2 Egg Whites, beaten very stiff
- 1/2 cup sugar, gradually added

- 1/2 t mint flavoring or almond extract
- 1/2 c. chocolate chips
- 1/4 cup chopped pecans
- food coloring

Directions

Preheat oven to 350. Beat eggs till very stiff. Gradually add sugar. Fold in last 3 ingredients. Also add food coloring in red or green. Cover cookie sheets with aluminum foil. Drop rounded tsp. slightly apart. Put in oven and TURN OFF the heat. Leave in closed oven at least 2 hours or overnight to dry up the cookies.

Number of Servings: 25

Spicy Chicken Breasts

Ingredients

- 2 ½ tablespoons paprika
- 2 tablespoons garlic powder
- 1 tablespoon salt
- 1 tablespoon onion powder
- 1 tablespoon dried thyme

- 1 tablespoon ground cayenne pepper
- 1 tablespoon ground black pepper
- 4 skinless, boneless chicken breast halves

Directions

In a medium bowl, mix together the paprika, garlic powder, salt, onion powder, thyme, cayenne pepper, and ground black pepper. Set aside about 3 tablespoons of this seasoning mixture for the chicken; store the remainder in an airtight container for later use (for seasoning fish, meats, or vegetables). Preheat grill for medium-high heat. Rub some of the reserved 3 tablespoons of seasoning onto both sides of the chicken breasts. Lightly oil the grill grate. Place chicken on the grill, and cook for 6 to 8 minutes on each side, until juices run clear.

Diet Soda Brownies

Ingredients

- 1 Box Brownie Mix
- 1/2 Can Diet Soda

Directions

Substitute the eggs, oil and water normally used in brownies for half a can of your favorite diet cola. Mix with the contents of store bought brownie mix. Make sure not to add anything to the mixture beside the half can of cola. Grease baking pan, poor in mixture and bake according to box.

Summer Tomato Casserole

Ingredients

- 6 vine ripened tomatoes, sliced
- 1 tablespoon mayonnaise (such as Hellman's®)
- 1 cup shredded Cheddar cheese
- salt and pepper to taste

Directions

Preheat oven to 350 degrees F (175 degrees C). Place a layer of tomato slices in an 8x8 inch baking pan. Spread a thin layer of mayonnaise on the tomatoes and sprinkle with about 1/4 of the Cheddar cheese and salt and pepper. Repeat layers, ending with the rest of the shredded cheese. Bake until tomatoes are softened and cheese is melted and bubbly, 20 to 25 minutes.

Sparkling Pomegranate Punch

Ingredients

- 3 cups pomegranate juice
- 3 cups orange juice
- 3 cups diet lemon-lime soda

Directions

First, make sure you have a pitcher large enough to hold 9 cups of liquid! Then pour everything together and gently stir. Garnish with mint. Makes nine 8 oz servings

Vegetable Masala

Servings: 4

Ingredients

- 2 potatoes, peeled and cubed
- 1 carrot, chopped
- 10 French-style green beans, chopped
- 1 quart cold water
- ½ cup frozen green peas, thawed

- 1 teaspoon salt
- ½ teaspoon ground turmeric
- 1 tablespoon vegetable oil
- 1 teaspoon mustard seed
- 1 teaspoon ground cumin
- 1 onion, finely chopped
- 2 tomatoes - blanched, peeled and chopped
- 1 teaspoon garam masala
- ½ teaspoon ground ginger
- ½ teaspoon garlic powder
- ½ teaspoon chili powder
- 1 sprig cilantro leaves, for garnish

Directions

Place potatoes, carrots and green beans in the cold water. Allow to soak while you prepare the rest of the vegetables; drain. In a microwave safe dish place the potatoes, carrots, green beans, peas, salt and turmeric. Cook for 8 minutes. Heat oil in a large skillet over medium heat. Cook mustard seeds and cumin; when seeds start to sputter and pop, add the onion and saute until transparent. Stir in the tomatoes, garam masala, ginger, garlic and chili powder; saute 3 minutes. Add the cooked vegetables to the tomato mixture and saute 1 minute. Garnish with cilantro leaves.

Shrimp Caesar Salad

Ingredients

- 2 Cups chopped Romaine lettuce fresh express hearts
- 1 Cup fresh Baby Spinach (raw)
- 1 Green Onion
- 8 halved Cherry Tomatoes, Fresh
- 1 Tbsp. Parmasan Grated Cheese
- 2 Tbsp. Cardini's Light Caesar Dressing 2 Tbsp
- 3 Shrimp, raw

Tips

I used cooked frozen shrimp. Nice because you can keep the bag frozen and take out a few shrimp here and there. They thaw quickly under cool running water. Then I removed the tail and cut up into bite size pieces with my kitchen shears.

Directions

Mix all ingredients up in a bowl and enjoy!

Serving Size: Makes 1 Serving

Number of Servings: 1

Chickpea Curry

Servings: 8

Ingredients

- 2 tablespoons vegetable oil
- 2 onions, minced
- 2 cloves garlic, minced
- 2 teaspoons fresh ginger root, finely chopped
- 6 whole cloves
- 2 (2 inch) sticks cinnamon, crushed
- 1 teaspoon ground cumin
- 1 teaspoon ground coriander
- salt
- 1 teaspoon cayenne pepper
- 1 teaspoon ground turmeric
- 2 (15 ounce) cans garbanzo beans

- 1 cup chopped fresh cilantro

Directions

Heat oil in a large frying pan over medium heat, and fry onions until tender. Stir in garlic, ginger, cloves, cinnamon, cumin, coriander, salt, cayenne, and turmeric. Cook for 1 minute over medium heat, stirring constantly. Mix in garbanzo beans and their liquid. Continue to cook and stir until all ingredients are well blended and heated through. Remove from heat. Stir in cilantro just before serving, reserving 1 tablespoon for garnish.

Christmas Punch

Ingredients

- 64 oz 100% Cranberry juice
- 2 liter Diet Sprite Zero
- 1 cup Cranberrie,s optional
- 2 limes
- ice

Directions

Pour cranberry juice and sprite into punch bowl. Then chop cranberries and slice limes. Add fruit to punch. Cover and chill. Add ice when ready to serve.

Authentic Tacos al Pastor

Servings: 10

Ingredients

- 1 tomato
- 3 dried guajillo chile peppers, seeded
- 2 dried ancho chile peppers, seeded
- 1 pineapple, sliced 3/4-inch thick
- ½ cup orange juice
- 1 onion, quartered
- ¼ cup white vinegar
- 2 chipotle peppers in adobo sauce
- 1 tablespoon salt, or to taste
- 2 cloves garlic, crushed
- 3 cloves

- 1 teaspoon cumin seeds
- 1 teaspoon dried oregano
- 2 pounds boneless pork loin, thinly sliced

To Serve:

- ½ cup chopped onion
- ½ cup chopped fresh cilantro

Directions

Cook tomato on a ridged grill pan over medium-high heat until slightly blackened, about 5 minutes. Remove from heat and cool until easily handled. Peel off skin and remove seeds. Bring a small pot of water to a boil. Add guajillo and ancho chile peppers; cook until softened, about 5 minutes. Drain. Combine tomato flesh, softened chile peppers, 2 slices pineapple, orange juice, quartered onion, vinegar, chipotle peppers, salt, garlic, cloves, cumin seeds, and oregano in a blender; blend until smooth. Arrange pork slices in a glass or ceramic baking dish. Pour blended mixture over pork, ensuring all sides are evenly coated. Cover baking dish with plastic wrap. Marinate pork in the refrigerator, 4 hours to overnight.

Cook remaining pineapple slices on a ridged grill pan over medium-high heat until slightly blackened and soft, about 5 minutes per side. Chop into small pieces. Wipe out grill pan and preheat over medium-high heat. Cook marinated pork in the hot pan, turning once, until browned, 4 to 5 minutes. Chop pork coarsely into small pieces against the grain. Serve with pineapple, chopped onion, and cilantro.

Mom's salad

Ingredients

- 2 heads romaine lettuce, thinly sliced
- 2 tomatoes, large diced
- 1 cucumber, large diced
- 1 red onion, thinly sliced
- 1/2 cup extra-virgin olive oil
- 1/4 cup red wine vinegar
- 2 tablespoons sour cream
- 1 teaspoon fresh oregano, chopped
- 1 clove garlic, minced
- Kosher salt and freshly cracked black pepper

Directions

Combine the romaine, tomatoes, cucumber and onions in a large bowl. Whisk the olive oil, vinegar, sour cream, oregano and garlic in a small bowl to make the vinaigrette. Pour the vinaigrette over the salad, season with salt and pepper and toss to combine. Serve with more freshly cracked black pepper over the top.

Old-Fashioned Vegetable Soup

Servings: 6

Ingredients

- 3 tablespoons butter
- 1 onion, diced
- 2 large carrots, diced
- 3 stalks celery, diced
- 1 (28 ounce) can whole peeled tomatoes, chopped, juice reserved
- 1 teaspoon salt
- ½ teaspoon ground black pepper

- 1 teaspoon dried parsley
- 3 tablespoons soy sauce
- 1 tablespoon Worcestershire sauce
- 1 teaspoon paprika
- 2 quarts beef broth

Directions

In a large pot over medium heat, melt butter. Cook onion, carrots and celery until onion is translucent. Stir in tomatoes with their juice, salt, pepper, parsley, soy sauce, Worcestershire and paprika. Pour in beef broth. Bring to a boil, then reduce heat and simmer 30 minutes, until vegetables are tender and flavors are well blended.

Sheet Pan Trifle

Ingredients

Cake:

- Nonstick baking spray, for the baking sheet
- 4 large eggs, cold
- 1 cup sugar
- 1 teaspoon baking powder

- 1 teaspoon kosher salt
- 1 stick (1/2 cup) unsalted butter, melted and cooled to room temperature
- 1 tablespoon pure vanilla extract
- 1 1/2 cups all-purpose flour, sifted

Assembly:

- 2 cups blackberries
- 2 cups blueberries
- 2 cups raspberries
- 2 cups strawberries, trimmed and quartered
- 2 tablespoons sugar
- 1 tablespoon finely grated lemon zest plus 1/4 cup lemon juice (from 1 lemon)
- 4 cups prepared instant lemon pudding
- 2 cups whipped cream

Directions

Special equipment: a 4-quart round trifle dish

For the cake: Position an oven rack in the center of the oven and preheat to 375 degrees F. Lightly coat an 18-by-

13-inch sheet pan with nonstick baking spray. Line the bottom with parchment. Set aside. Beat the eggs, sugar, baking powder and salt in a stand mixer fitted with the whisk attachment on high speed until the mixture is pale and very thick (enough to hold a wake from whisk), about 10 minutes. Reduce the speed to medium-high and drizzle in the butter and vanilla until just combined, about 10 seconds. Reduce the speed to low and add the sifted flour all at once. Beat until just combined, about 5 seconds. Gently fold the batter once or twice using a rubber spatula, then scrape it into the prepared sheet pan. Spread it evenly with the spatula, using broad, gentle strokes to keep the batter airy. Bake, rotating the pan halfway through, until the top is lightly golden, 15 to 18 minutes. Cool in the sheet pan for 10 minutes, then invert onto a wire rack and cool completely. For the assembly: Combine the blackberries, blueberries, raspberries, and strawberries with the sugar and lemon zest and juice in a large bowl and lightly toss with a spoon to combine. Set aside for 15 minutes to allow the berries to release some juice. Use a sharp paring knife to cut out 2 rounds and 2 half-rounds from the sheet cake, using the top of the trifle dish as a guide. The 2 half-circles can be combined to create 1 whole circle. This gives you 3 layers of cake. Reserve all the cake scraps.

Spread about 1 1/3 cups of the lemon pudding in the bottom of a 4-quart round trifle dish, then top with a cake round, about 2 cups of berries (including some of the juices) and about 1/2 cup of the whipped cream. Repeat the layers 2 more times. Pile the remaining berries on top in the center and spread the remaining whipped cream around the edges. Crumble there rerved scraps of cake with your fingers and sprinkle over the whipped cream.

Mediterranean Tilapia

Servings: 2

Ingredients

- 3 tablespoons sun-dried tomatoes packed in oil, drained and chopped
- 1 tablespoon capers, drained
- 2 tilapia fillets
- 1 tablespoon oil from the jar of sun dried tomatoes

- 1 tablespoon lemon juice
- 2 tablespoons kalamata olives, pitted and chopped

Directions

Preheat the oven to 375 degrees F (190 degrees C). In a small bowl, stir together the sun-dried tomatoes, olives and capers. Set aside. Place the tilapia fillets side by side in a baking dish. Drizzle with oil and lemon juice. Bake for 10 to 15 minutes in the preheated oven, until the fish flakes with a fork. Check after 10 minutes, so as not to overcook, or the fish may be dry. When fish is done, top with the tomato mixture, and serve.

Whole Roasted Sweet Potatoes

Ingredients

- Four 8-ounce sweet potatoes
- Extra-virgin olive oil, for rubbing and drizzling
- Kosher salt and freshly ground black pepper
- Shaved Parmesan, for serving

Directions

Preheat the oven to 425 degrees F. Wash the potatoes well and pat dry. Poke holes all around each potato using a fork. Rub the potatoes all over with oil, then sprinkle liberally with salt and pepper. Place the potatoes on a baking sheet or aluminum foil and roast until tender when pierced with a fork, 40 to 45 minutes. Transfer the potatoes to a plate and serve with shaved Parmesan and a drizzle of olive oil.

Italian Leafy Green Salad

Servings: 6

Yield: 6 1-cup servings

Ingredients

- 2 cups romaine lettuce - torn, washed and dried
- 1 cup torn escarole
- 1 cup torn radicchio
- 1 cup torn red leaf lettuce
- ¼ cup chopped green onions

- ½ red bell pepper, sliced into rings
- ½ green bell pepper, sliced in rings
- 12 cherry tomatoes
- ¼ cup grapeseed oil
- 2 tablespoons chopped fresh basil
- ¼ cup balsamic vinegar
- 2 tablespoons lemon juice
- salt and pepper to taste

Directions

In a large bowl, combine the romaine, escarole, radicchio, red-leaf, scallions, red pepper, green pepper and cherry tomatoes. Whisk together the grapeseed oil, basil, vinegar, lemon juice and salt and pepper. Pour over salad, toss and serve immediately.

Vegan chickpea crab cakes

Ingredients

Chickpea Crab Cakes:

- Two 15-ounce cans chickpeas, drained and 1/4 cup liquid reserved

- Pinch cream of tartar
- 2 tablespoons fresh parsley, chopped
- 1 tablespoon lemon juice, plus lemon wedges for serving
- 2 teaspoons Old Bay Seasoning
- 1 teaspoon honey mustard
- 2 slices of white bread or 1 hamburger bun, torn into small pieces
- Kosher salt
- 2/3 cup all-purpose flour
- Vegetable oil, for frying

Tartar Sauce:

- 1/4 cup vegan mayonnaise
- 1/2 teaspoon honey mustard
- Pinch Old Bay Seasoning
- 1/2 whole dill pickle, finely chopped
- 1 tablespoon dill pickle brine

Directions

For the chickpea crab cakes: Place the reserved chickpea liquid into a large bowl, then add the cream of tartar and whip vigorously until foamy and thick. Whisk in the parsley, lemon juice, Old Bay and honey mustard, then add the bread pieces and toss to coat. Let sit until the bread is soft, about 5 minutes. Meanwhile, finely chop the chickpeas (alternatively, you can pinch or smush them). When the bread mixture is ready, add the chickpeas and toss and squeeze the mixture until it holds together. Form into eight 3/4-inch thick patties with nice rounded edges. Cover and chill them for at least 1 hour.

For the tartar sauce: Whisk together the mayonnaise, honey mustard, Old Bay, pickle and pickle brine in a small bowl. Refrigerate until ready to serve.

Preheat the oven to 350 degrees F. Whisk a large pinch of salt into the flour and put on a plate. Pour enough oil to cover the bottom of a large nonstick skillet and heat over medium-high heat. Dredge half of the cakes in the flour. Once the oil is hot and shimmering, add the cakes and cook until crunchy and deep golden brown, about 3 minutes per side. Adjust the heat as necessary to keep them from browning too quickly. Transfer to a baking sheet and repeat with the remaining cakes. Sprinkle each with salt, then bake until heated completely through, about 5 minutes. Serve the chickpea crab cakes with the tartar sauce and lemon wedges.

Blueberry Walnut Salad

Servings: 6

Yield: 6 servings

Ingredients

- 1 (10 ounce) package mixed salad greens
- 1 pint fresh blueberries
- ¼ cup walnuts
- ½ cup raspberry vinaigrette salad dressing
- ¼ cup crumbled feta cheese

Directions

In a large bowl, toss the salad greens with the blueberries, walnuts, and raspberry vinaigrette. Top with feta cheese to serve.

Simple Boiled Broccoli

Ingredients

- 1 bunch broccoli (about 1 pound)
- Kosher salt and freshly ground black pepper
- Lemon wedges, for serving

Directions

Wash the broccoli in cold water and pat dry. Peel the stem and trim right where the florets branch off. Break apart the florets. Bring a pot of salted water to a boil. Add the broccoli florets and cook, uncovered, until tender, 2 to 3 minutes depending on the size of the florets. Drain into a colander, transfer to a plate, sprinkle with salt and pepper and serve with lemon wedges.

Wonderful Raspberry Walnut Dinner Salad

Servings: 5

Yield: 5 servings

Ingredients

- 1 (10 ounce) package mixed salad greens, rinsed and dried
- 1 (8 ounce) package sweetened dried cranberries
- ¼ cup sunflower seeds
- 4 roma (plum) tomatoes, chopped
- 1 avocado - peeled, pitted and diced
- ½ (8 ounce) bottle raspberry walnut vinaigrette

Directions

In a large bowl, toss together the salad greens, cranberries, sunflower seeds and tomatoes. Top with avocado (and chicken strips, if desired), add vinaigrette and serve.

Mustard-Parmesan Whole Roasted Cauliflower

Ingredients

- 2 large heads cauliflower
- 1 clove garlic, halved
- 1/4 cup olive oil
- 4 tablespoons Dijon mustard

- Kosher salt and freshly ground black pepper
- 1/2 cup fresh parsley leaves, roughly chopped
- 1/4 cup grated Parmesan
- Lemon wedges, for serving

Directions

Position an oven rack in the bottom of the oven and preheat to 450 degrees F. Line a baking sheet with foil. Remove the leaves from the cauliflower, then trim the stem flush with the bottom of the head so the cauliflower sits flat on the prepared baking sheet. Rub the outside of each head with the cut garlic. Whisk together the oil, 3 tablespoons mustard, 1/2 teaspoon salt and a few grinds of black pepper in a small bowl. Put the cauliflower on the prepared baking sheet and brush the entire outside and inside with the mustard-oil mixture. Roast the cauliflower until nicely charred and tender (a long skewer inserted in the center of the cauliflower should pass through easily), 50 minutes to 1 hour. Let rest for a few minutes. Meanwhile, combine the parsley and Parmesan in a small bowl. Brush the outside of the roasted cauliflower heads all over with the remaining 1 tablespoon mustard and generously sprinkle with the Parmesan mixture. Cut the cauliflower into thick wedges and serve on plates with a sprinkle of salt, lemon wedges and any extra Parmesan mixture.

Greens and Beans

Servings: 8

Yield: 8 servings

Ingredients

- 1 teaspoon salt
- 2 heads escarole, cut into 2-inch pieces
- ¼ cup olive oil
- 3 cloves garlic, pressed
- 1 teaspoon salt, or more to taste
- ½ teaspoon black pepper
- ¼ teaspoon red pepper flakes
- 1 (15 ounce) can cannellini beans, drained and rinsed
- 1 tablespoon Parmesan cheese, or to taste (Optional)

Directions

Pour enough water into a large pot to be about 2 inches deep; bring to a boil. Stir 1 teaspoon salt into the boiling water; add escarole. Cook the escarole at a boil, pushing the escarole further into the water as it wilts, until it is fork-tender, 3 to 5 minutes; drain. Pour olive oil into the pot and place over medium heat. Cook and stir garlic, 1 teaspoon salt, black pepper, and red pepper flakes in hot oil until the garlic is soft, 3 to 5 minutes. Stir drained escarole and cannellini beans into the garlic mixture; cook and stir until the beans are hot, 5 to 10 minutes. Sprinkle Parmesan cheese over the mixture just before serving.

15-Minute Shrimp Tacos with Spicy Chipotle Slaw

Ingredients

- 1 pound medium (26/30) peeled and deveined shrimp, tails removed
- 2 teaspoons chili powder
- Kosher salt
- 2 tablespoons canola oil

- 4 scallions, thinly sliced
- One 15-ounce can black beans, drained and rinsed well
- 1/3 cup prepared chipotle mayonnaise
- 2 limes, 1 zested and juiced and 1 cut into wedges
- One 14-ounce bag store-bought coleslaw mix (about 6 cups)
- 1 bunch fresh cilantro, leaves and soft stems roughly chopped
- Sour cream or Mexican crema, for serving
- 8 corn tortillas, warmed

Directions

Heat a large cast-iron skillet over medium-high heat. Combine the shrimp, chili powder and a large pinch of salt in a medium bowl and stir to combine. Add the canola oil to the hot skillet and swirl to coat. Add the shrimp and cook until the shrimp is no longer opaque and just cooked through, turning only once, about 2 minutes. Transfer the shrimp to a serving bowl and cover loosely with foil to keep warm. Stir 2 tablespoons of water into the skillet with the dripping, using a wooden spoon or heat-proof spatula to scrape up any browned bits at the bottom of the skillet. Reserve 1 tablespoon scallions for garnish and add the rest to the skillet. Cook until the scallions are slightly softened, stirring frequently, about 1 minute. Add the beans and a large pinch of salt and cook until warmed through, about 1 minute. Turn off the heat and reserve. In a large bowl, stir together the chipotle mayonnaise, lime zest and juice and a large pinch of salt. Add the coleslaw mix and half of the cilantro and stir to combine. Serve the shrimp alongside the beans, coleslaw, remaining cilantro, scallions, sour cream or Mexican crema, lime wedges and warm tortillas.

Fish on a Plank

Servings: 6

Yield: 6 servings

Ingredients

- 1 cedar plank
- 6 (5 ounce) mahi mahi fillets
- 1 cup bottled teriyaki sauce
- 2 mangos - peeled, seeded and diced

- ½ red bell pepper, seeded and chopped
- 4 green onions, chopped
- 1 tablespoon chopped fresh cilantro
- 1 jalapeno pepper, seeded and chopped
- salt and pepper to taste
- ½ teaspoon garlic powder
- 1 teaspoon fresh lime juice
- 1 teaspoon lemon juice
- 2 teaspoons olive oil
- 1 teaspoon chipotle seasoning
- 1 teaspoon red pepper flakes
- 1 teaspoon hot-pepper sauce

Directions

In a medium bowl, combine the mangos, bell pepper, green onion, cilantro and jalapeno pepper. Season with salt, pepper, garlic powder and lime juice. Stir together then cover and refrigerate until serving to blend the flavors. Soak the plank in water for at least 2 hours, longer if possible. Place the mahi mahi fillets in a shallow dish and coat with teriyaki sauce. Cover, and marinate for at least 1 hour. Prepare a grill for indirect heat. If using charcoal, arrange and light coals under one half of the grill. Sprinkle lemon juice over the fish fillets and season with chipotle seasoning, red pepper flakes and hot pepper sauce. Place the fillets on the plank. Place the plank on the grill over direct heat. Cover and cook for 10 minutes. Move the plank with the fish over to indirect heat (the cooler part of the grill), cover and cook for 10 more minutes or until fish can be flaked with a fork. Top fillets with mango salsa and serve hot.

Deep Dish Quiche with Garnishes

Ingredients

- All-purpose flour (for surface)
- 2 shallots, finely chopped
- 2 Tbsp. extra-virgin olive oil
- 1 1/2 tsp. kosher salt, divided
- 1 Tbsp. finely chopped chives
- 8 large eggs
- 1 3/4 cups half-and-half
- 1/2 tsp. freshly ground black pepper
- 1 cup crème fraîche, plus more for serving

Braised Leeks, Peas, and Lettuce, prosciutto or other cured meat and/or salmon, green goddess dressing, avocado, baby greens, and lemon wedges (for serving)

Directions

Roll dough to a 15" round on a lightly floured work surface; trim edges. Fit dough into a 9" springform pan, letting dough fold over itself slightly around the edges so that it creates a gently pleated, rippled effect (the dough will extend above top of pan). Place pan on a rimmed baking sheet. Chill 1 hour, or freeze 20 minutes. Preheat oven to 350°F. Dock bottom surface of dough with a fork. Line dough with parchment paper or foil, then fill with dried beans or baking weights. Bake crust on baking sheet until top edge is golden, about 30 minutes. Using parchment, lift out beans, then continue to bake until surface of crust is set and lightly browned and feels dry, 35–40 minutes more. Transfer pan to a wire rack and let cool. While crust cools, reduce oven temperature to 325°F. Cook shallots, oil, and 1/2 tsp. salt in a small skillet over medium-low heat, stirring often, until tender and translucent, about 5 minutes. Remove from heat and stir in chives. Spoon filling into cooled crust. Vigorously whisk eggs in a large bowl or glass measuring cup. Whisk in half-and-half, pepper, 1 cup crème fraîche, and remaining 1 tsp. salt until combined. Pour custard over filling. Bake quiche until filling is puffed, set, and golden, 60–75 minutes. Transfer pan to a wire rack and let cool at least 1 hour. Release springform, then lift quiche off base using parchment overhang and transfer to a platter or cutting board. Serve with braised vegetables, prosciutto, crème fraîche, green goddess dressing, avocado, greens, and lemon wedges alongside for guests to dress their quiche as desired.

Do Ahead: Crust can be baked 1 day ahead. Store uncovered at room temperature. Quiche can be made 6 hours ahead. Store uncovered at room temperature. Quiche can also be made 1 day ahead; cover and chill overnight. Bring to room temperature 2 hours before serving.

Birria Recipe

Servings: 12

Yield: 12 servings

Ingredients

- 5 dried Anaheim chile peppers, stemmed and seeded
- 5 guajillo chile peppers, stemmed and seeded
- water to cover
- ¼ onion
- 1 tablespoon mixed spices, or more to taste
- 1 tablespoon salt, or to taste
- 3 pounds cubed beef stew meat
- 6 bay leaves

Directions

Place Anaheim and guajillo peppers in a saucepan and cover with water; bring to a boil. Reduce heat to medium-low and simmer until tender, about 15 minutes. Remove saucepan from heat and cool for 5 minutes. Pour chiles and water into a blender; add onion, mixed spices, and salt. Blend until sauce is smooth. Mix stew meat, sauce, and bay leaves in a large pot; cook over medium-low heat until meat is very tender, 3 to 5 hours.

Tip

Aluminum foil helps keep food moist, ensures it cooks evenly, keeps leftovers fresh, and makes clean-up easy.

Goat Cheese Stuffed Peppadews

Ingredients

- 6 ounces soft goat cheese, room temperature
- 2 large garlic cloves, minced
- 2 tablespoons chopped fresh basil, chives, thyme, or other fresh herbs
- 2 tablespoons heavy cream or half-and-half (as needed)
- salt and pepper, to taste
- 1 jar peppadew peppers (about 20-30 peppers)

Directions

In a bowl, combine goat cheese with garlic and herbs, stirring until evenly incorporated. Add cream as needed, 1 tablespoon at a time, to thin out filling if necessary (the amount needed will depend mostly on the softness of your goat cheese). The filling should be the consistency of buttercream frosting. Season to taste with salt and pepper.

Fill each peppadew with about 1/2 teaspoon of filling. I find it helpful to load the filling into a piping bag fitted with a 1/4-inch round tip, which makes it very easy to neatly fill each pepper completely full. Serve immediately or refrigerate for up to 2 hours; let come to room temperature for 15 minutes prior to serving.

Shrimp Taco Bites

These quick and easy Shrimp Taco Bites are the perfect appetizer for parties or entertaining!

Ingredients

- 24 large raw shrimps, peels and tails removed
- non-stick cooking spray, or olive oil spray
- 1 tsp salt, divided
- 1 tsp lime zest, grated(+ juice 1 tbsp lime juice)
- 2 tsp chili powder
- 1 large California Avocado, diced
- 1/3 cup sour cream
- 1 tsp chipotle chilies in adobo sauce, finely minced
- 2 tbsp chopped cilantro, fresh

- 24 to tortilla chip scoops
- US Customary - Metric

Directions

Pre heat oven to 375 degrees F. Spray a large baking sheet or cookie sheet with non-stick cooking spray or olive oil spray, set aside. Combine 1/2 tsp salt, lime zest, and chili powder in a small bowl. Sprinkle all over the raw shrimp. Lay the shrimp on the cookie sheet and spritz with the non stick cooking spray or olive oil spray. Bake for 5-8 minutes or until the shrimps turn pink and curl in on themselves. Meanwhile combine the diced avocado, lime juice and remaining 1/2 tsp salt in a small bowl. Combine the sour cream and minced chipotle pepper in a different small bowl. Assemble your shrimp taco bites by placing a tsp of avocado mixture in a tortilla chip, followed by a 1/2 tsp of sour cream mixture, then top with a chili-lime shrimp. Sprinkle with the chopped cilantro. Enjoy!

Notes

These bites are best when prepared just before serving.

Prosciutto & Fresh Mozzarella on Grilled Garlic Toasts

Ingredients

- 1 baguette
- 2 cloves of garlic, peeled
- 3 tablespoons of olive oil
- 8 ounces of fresh mozzarella, sliced
- 6 slices of prosciutto, thinly sliced
- sea salt & cracked pepper
- fresh basil, chopped

Directions

Prepare the bread by slicing into thin slices. Grill bread just before serving. You can do it under the broiler in your oven, or on the grill. Brush the bread with olive oil on one side. If broiling, place them on a sheet oiled side up and place them under the broiler for 1-2 minutes. Be careful not to burn! If grilling, also grill the bread for 1-2 minutes. When you remove them from the grill or oven, let them cool slightly, then rub the raw clove of garlic on each piece. If grilling, brush the other side of the bread with oil, then put that side down on the baking sheet or tray. If you are broiling in the oven, just keep the toasts on the sheet with their toasted side up. Top each piece of bread with small, thin slices of prosciutto. Then, top each with a slice of fresh mozzarella. Grill or broil the toasts for 2 minutes, or just until the mozzarella begins to melt. Remove from the grill or broiler and top with salt, pepper and fresh basil. Ready to go on the grill along with some artichokes. The toasts have been grilled, now I'm ready to top them with prosciutto and cheese.

Smashed Sweet Potato Guacamole Bites

These smashed sweet potato guacamole bites have crispy sides with soft centers. Topped with a crispy piece of salty bacon, they're the perfect game day bite.

Ingredients

- 3 medium sweet potatoes
- extra virgin olive oil
- salt and pepper
- 2 avocados
- juice of 1/2 a lime
- 1 clove garlic, minced

- 1/2 jalapeno, minced
- 1/4 cup chopped cilantro
- 3 slices bacon, cooked

Directions

Clean sweet potatoes leaving skin on. Place in a large pot and cover with water. Boil potatoes for about 20 minutes until tender. Preheat oven to 450 degrees. Remove potatoes from water, slice into thick rounds (about 1/2 inch) and place on a greased baking sheet. Using a fork, gently smash the tops of the potatoes. Drizzle the potato rounds with olive oil and season liberally with salt and pepper. Place potatoes in the oven for 20-22 minutes until the edges are crispy and starting to turn golden brown. While potatoes cook, combine the avocados, lime juice, garlic, jalapeno and cilantro in a small bowl. Mash together until smooth. Chop the bacon into 1/2 inch pieces and set aside. Remove the potatoes from the oven, top with a spoonful of the guacamole and a piece of bacon. Serve warm.

ESPN Zone's Spinach and Artichoke Dip

Ingredients

Spinach and Artichoke Dip

- 4 tablespoons (1/2 stick) butter
- 1/4 cup diced onion
- 3 cloves garlic, minced
- 1/4 cup all-purpose flour
- 1 cup heavy cream
- 2 cups whole or 2% milk
- 1/8 teaspoon white pepper
- 2 1/2 cups grated Parmesan cheese
- 1 teaspoon coarse salt
- 1 teaspoon freshly ground black pepper
- 2 teaspoons Worcestershire sauce
- 2 teaspoons hot sauce, such as Tabasco
- 8-ounce package cream cheese, cut into cubes and softened
- 2 1/2 (10-ounce) boxes frozen chopped spinach, thawed and squeezed dry

- 2 (14.5-ounce) cans quartered artichoke hearts, drained
- 1 cup shredded mozzarella
- Tortilla chips, carrot and celery sticks, garlic bread, for serving

Directions

Preheat oven to 350°F. Melt butter in a large stockpot over medium heat. Add onions and garlic and sauté 2 minutes. Add flour; cook for 4 minutes, stirring constantly. Slowly whisk in cream and milk, then bring to simmer, whisking often until sauce is thick and coats the back of a spoon. Add white pepper and Parmesan, stirring until well incorporated. Remove from heat. Add salt, pepper, Worcestershire, and hot sauce. Mix well. Fold in cream cheese, stirring well until cream cheese is completely incorporated. Add spinach, stirring to combine. Add artichoke hearts, stirring gently so as not to break up the artichokes. Pour mixture into a 9×9-inch baking dish and sprinkle mozzarella evenly on top. Bake 15 minutes, or until cheese on top is completely melted and bubbling. Serve hot with tortilla chips, carrot and celery sticks, and/or garlic bread

Watermelon Fruit Bowl

Servings: 20

Yield: 20 servings

Ingredients

- 1 large watermelon
- 1 cantaloupe, halved and seeded
- 1 honeydew melon, halved and seeded
- 2 (15 ounce) cans mandarin oranges, drained
- 2 (20 ounce) cans pineapple chunks, drained
- 2 cups halved fresh strawberries
- 2 cups seedless grapes
- ½ cup water
- ¼ cup white sugar
- 2 tablespoons grated lemon zest

Directions

With a large, sharp knife, remove the top 1/4 section of the watermelon. With a melon baller, scoop flesh from inside of watermelon, removing as many seeds as possible. Leave 1/2 inch of flesh inside the shell of the watermelon. Scoop cantaloupe and honeydew in the same manner, removing as much flesh as possible, and discarding the rinds. Refrigerate fruits separately until ready to assemble. In a small saucepan over medium-high heat, bring water and sugar to a boil. Remove from heat, and continue stirring until sugar has completely dissolved. Add lemon zest, and set aside to cool. To serve, place watermelon balls, cantaloupe, honeydew, oranges, pineapple, strawberries, and grapes, in a large mixing bowl. Pour syrup over, and toss thoroughly. Transfer mixture to watermelon bowl, and serve. Set aside any fruit mixture that will not fit. There will be enough fruit to refill the bowl.

CONCLUSION

While the amount of weight you will lose on a diet plan depends on a number of factors, including your starting weight, your gender, your activity level, etc. Most experts recommend a steady weight loss of one to two pounds per week, since studies suggest that those who lose weight gradually and steadily are more successful at keeping it off. When you're shopping for a healthy diet plan for weight loss, you'll want to keep this in mind. Companies that force you to follow an 800 calorie diet plan, or promise that you'll lose weight fast—like 20 pounds in a few days, are not only unhealthy, they're not sustainable. Opt for a weight loss program that promises steady weight loss, and you'll set yourself up for long-term success.

www.ingramcontent.com/pod-product-compliance
Lightning Source LLC
LaVergne TN
LVHW010501160826
845677LV00012B/2600

* 9 7 9 8 3 5 5 4 6 8 6 8 2 *